I0454476

# THE PERFECT ACID REFLUX DIET

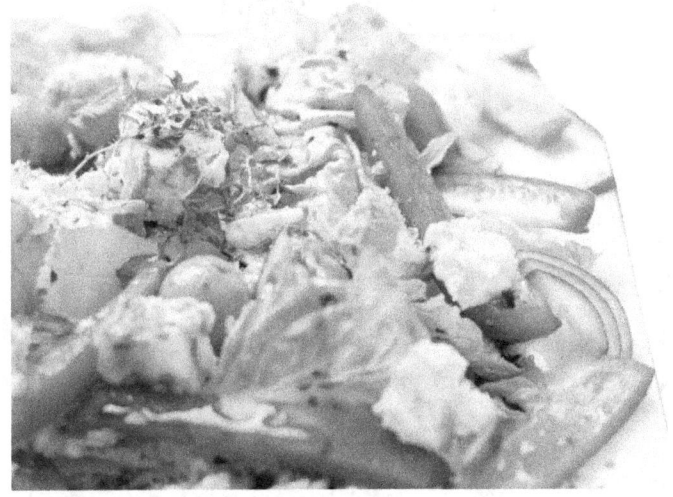

*A Complete Cookbook for Beginners for Crafting the Ideal Diet for Perfect Digestive Harmony*

Isabelle Hartley

i

**Copyright © 2023 By [ Isabelle Hartley]**

**All content in this book is protected under copyright laws. Any reproduction, distribution, or unauthorized use of any part of this book without the prior written consent of the copyright owner is strictly prohibited except for personal use.**

# OTHER BOOKS BY THIS AUTHOR

1. GASTROPARESIS DIET RECIPES COOKBOOK
2. HIGH CALORIES DIET COOKBOOK
3. DIET FOR WOMEN OVER FORTY
4. HASHIMOTO RECIPES COOKBOOK
5. JUICING RECIPES FOR CANCER
6. IVF DIET COOKBOOK FOR BEGINNERS
7. LOW SUGAR DIET GUIDE FOR BEGINNERS
8. RAW FOODS RECIPES COOKBOOK
9. SMOOTHIES RECIPES FOR ANTI-INFLAMMATION
10. MEDITERRANEAN DIET FOR PREGNANT WOMEN

# TABLE OF CONTENTS

# Introduction

Allow me to start this book with the story of Mrs. Thompson, an old woman whose laughter could be heard all over the streets but whose joy was tempered by her ongoing struggle with acid reflux. Even though she was full of life, the pain had become a lifelong friend, lowering her mood.

As luck would have it, a young couple who were interested in getting to know everyone in the community moved in next door one day. Emma and Jack saw Mrs. Thompson's unease as they conversed casually across the fence. They were worried and decided to look into it in order to assist her in getting better.

Equipped with an education and a love of cooking, Emma set off on a culinary adventure. She devoted endless hours to developing recipes designed to reduce the symptoms of acid reflux. Excited to share her discoveries, she knocked on Mrs. Thompson's door with her prepared delicacies in hand.

Mrs. Thompson accepted Emma's kind offer and tasted the food with a mixture of optimism and mistrust. She was surprised that the thoughtfully prepared meals didn't cause her typical pain. Gradually, the pain subsided and her happiness reappeared like a lost tune.

There was a notable change in the neighborhood. Mrs. Thompson laughed hesitantly at first, but suddenly it rang with true joy. Everyone was captivated by her sudden vitality as it radiated through the streets. Emma and Jack were gratified to see their neighbor's amazing recovery.

Mrs. Thompson made the decision to create a cookbook using Emma's recipes after being inspired by her travels. The publication of "The Perfect Acid Reflux Diet Cookbook" was the result of a neighbor's desire for treatment and another person's generosity. It became a ray of hope for countless others struggling with related problems, a practical manual for recovering happiness and comfort with mindful eating.

The community rejoiced in Mrs. Thompson's new lease on life as well as the priceless relationship that resulted from a straightforward gesture of care.

# CHAPTER 1

## About this book

Introducing "The Perfect Acid Reflux Diet," a carefully curated gastronomic adventure designed to soothe and relieve people attempting to control or even reverse the difficulties associated with acid reflux. In a world where food decisions significantly impact our health, this cookbook seeks to serve as your reliable guide toward digestive balance.

The backflow of stomach acid into the esophagus, or acid reflux, can cause significant disruptions to day-to-day functioning. Its symptoms affect people of all ages and vary from the burning sensation of heartburn to more serious consequences. Understanding that you require a comprehensive strategy, this cookbook has been carefully selected to provide you with tasty fixes that will both calm and nourish you.

We start our adventure by learning about the subtleties of acid reflux and the things that might cause it. You will have a thorough understanding of the foods that can alleviate this disease as well as those that contribute to it through enlightening advice and suggestions. This information serves as the cornerstone of our recipe collection, which is motivated by the goal of offering both gastronomic delight and healthful advantages.

"The Perfect Acid Reflux Diet" goes beyond the idea of a restricted diet. It encourages you to try a wide variety of mouthwatering recipes that follow the guidelines of a diet that is beneficial to acid reflux sufferers. Every recipe, from colorful salads to filling main courses and decadent desserts, is proof that enjoying great meals shouldn't have to be sacrificed in order to control acid reflux.

This cookbook is a lifestyle guide that promotes thoughtful choices that align with your body's requirements, rather than just a collection of recipes. May you have relief from acid reflux symptoms as well as a renewed appreciation for the art of providing your body with delicious, health-conscious food as you set out on this culinary adventure. Greetings from a universe where healthful digestion and deliciousness coexist.

## Gastroesophageal Reflux Disease

Gastritis reflux disease (GERD), also referred to as acid reflux disease, is a chronic illness that arises when stomach acid continuously runs back into the esophagus. The esophagus lining may become irritated and inflamed due to this frequent acid reflux, which may result in a variety of symptoms and possible consequences. Comprehending the many forms, origins, and indications of acid reflux is vital for efficient handling and avoidance.

### Acid reflux types:

The most prevalent kind of GERD is called Non-Erosive Reflux Disease (NERD), which is characterized by reflux symptoms that are normal but do not show any visible damage to the esophageal lining during endoscopy.

This kind of erosive esophagitis is caused by frequent exposure to stomach acid and manifests as apparent damage to the esophagus. From minor irritation to severe inflammation and ulceration, it can range in severity.

- Barrett's Esophagus: Barrett's esophagus is a more severe GERD problem in which the lining of the esophagus changes as a result of prolonged exposure to stomach acid. The risk of esophageal cancer is elevated in individuals with this disease.
- Acid reflux causes include: Lower Sphincter of the Esophagus (LES) Dysfunction: The ring of muscle that divides the stomach and esophagus is called the LES. Reflux can result from stomach acid flowing back into the esophagus when it doesn't seal correctly.
- Hiatal Hernia: When a piece of the stomach pushes through the diaphragm, it causes a hiatal hernia, which interferes with the LES's regular operation and aggravates acid reflux.
- Dietary factors: A number of foods and drinks, including chocolate, tomatoes, citrus fruits, coffee, and spicy or fatty meals, can

cause or exacerbate symptoms of acid reflux.

- Obesity: Carrying too much weight, especially in the abdominal region, can raise intra-abdominal pressure and push stomach acid down the esophagus.

- Pregnancy: Acid reflux symptoms may arise as a result of hormonal changes and increased abdominal pressure.

- Smoking: Smoking weakens the LES and is a factor in acid reflux development.

## Signs of acid reflux include:

The most typical symptom is heartburn, which is defined by a burning feeling in the chest that can spread to the neck. It usually happens when you're lying down or after eating.

- Regurgitation: The reflux of stomach contents into the mouth, frequently with an aftertaste that is bitter or sour.

- Dysphagia: Trouble swallowing, which might be a sign of more serious esophageal injury.
- Chest Pain: A pain in the chest that may resemble the signs of a heart attack. It's critical to distinguish between cardiac problems and chest pain brought on by acid reflux.
- Chronic Cough: Acid reflux that irritates the airways can cause a chronic cough, especially at night.
- Hoarseness or a raspy voice can be caused by laryngitis, an inflammation of the voice box.
- Acid reflux: This condition might exacerbate asthma episodes or asthma symptoms.
- Dental Issues: Dental issues may arise from tooth enamel erosion brought on by acid exposure.

Diagnose and Therapy:

**Diagnostic Examinations:**

Endoscopy: A technique to check for injury to the esophagus.

pH monitoring: Determines the frequency and duration of acid reflux by measuring the esophageal acidity levels over time.

Manometry: Assesses the LES's operation and pressure.

**Changes in Lifestyle:**

Modifications to Diet: Steer clear of trigger foods and choose a diet high in non-fatty, low-acid, and non-spicy meals.

Weight control: Reducing extra weight helps ease the strain on the abdomen.

Raising the Head of the Bed: Sleeping with the upper torso raised might aid in avoiding acid reflux.

**Drugs:**

- Antacids: By neutralizing stomach acid, they offer immediate relief.
- H2 Blockers: Diminish gastric acid production.
- Proton pump inhibitors (PPIs): Prevent the generation of acid and aid in esophageal repair.
- Surgery: To strengthen the LES in extreme situations or when other therapies are ineffective, surgical alternatives such fundoplication may be taken into consideration.

**Lifestyle Modifications to Control Acid Reflux:**

- Meal Timing: Eating more often and in smaller portions might assist avoid filling up the stomach.
- Eliminating Trigger meals: The key to controlling acid reflux symptoms is recognizing and avoiding meals and drinks that cause symptoms.

- Sustaining a Healthy Weight: Reducing abdominal pressure can be accomplished by reaching and maintaining a healthy weight.

- Posture and Sleeping Position: To lessen the chance of acid reflux, keep your back straight after eating and raise your head before you go to bed. Quitting Smoking: Smoking weakens the LES, therefore giving it up is good for your general health and the treatment of acid reflux.

In summary, acid reflux is a common and frequently chronic ailment that necessitates a multimodal approach to treatment. Those looking for treatment and hoping to avoid consequences must understand its forms, causes, and symptoms. By treating acid reflux, one can enhance quality of life and lower the chance of long-term consequences. This can be achieved by lifestyle changes, medication, or, in extreme circumstances, surgical treatments. It is best to speak with a healthcare provider if you think you may have acid reflux in order to receive an accurate diagnosis and customized treatment recommendations.

# CHAPTER 2

## Foods To Eat or Avoid on Acid Reflux Diet

Making thoughtful food selections is part of following an acid reflux diet that can help reduce symptoms and encourage digestive comfort. The idea is to lessen the possibility that stomach acid would reflux back into the esophagus, which will lessen the likelihood of heartburn, regurgitation, and other related discomforts. This is a thorough advice on what foods to put on and take off an acid reflux diet:

## Foods to Consume: Fruits That Are Not Citrus

Choose fruits that are less acidic and less prone to cause reflux symptoms, such as bananas, apples, and pears.

Produce: Vegetables are often well accepted. Broccoli, cauliflower, potatoes, and green leafy vegetables are good options. Steer clear of using too much oil or butter when preparing.

Trim Proteins: Select lean protein sources including fish, chicken, and lean meat cuts. It is better to grill, bake, or simmer these proteins instead of frying them.

Complete Grains: Add healthful grains such as quinoa, brown rice, and oatmeal. They give you fiber, which promotes good digestion and weight management.

Dairy products: Select dairy products that are fat-free or low-fat. You can include milk, yogurt, and certain cheeses in your diet, but you should always keep an eye on your own tolerance.

Spices and Herbs: Ginger, oregano, and fennel are examples of mild herbs and spices that may be used to boost taste without being too acidic.

Good Fats: Add foods like avocados, almonds, and olive oil that are good sources of fat. Unlike trans or saturated fats, these fats are less prone to cause acid reflux.

Uncaffeinated Drinks: Sip herbal teas, water, and non-citrus, non-mint flavored drinks. It can help with digestion and is important for general health to stay hydrated.

Ginger: Ginger, which has anti-inflammatory qualities, may help relieve gastrointestinal discomfort. It may be eaten in a variety of ways, such as a spice in food or in ginger tea.

Aloe Vera Juice: When taken in moderation, aloe vera juice can help soothe inflamed esophageal tissues.

## Foods to Steer Clear of:
Fruits with Citrus Flavors: Due to their high acidity, oranges, grapefruits, lemons, and other citrus fruits can make acid reflux symptoms worse. Choose non-citrus substitutes.

Tomatoes: Due to their acidic nature, tomatoes and tomato-based products such as sauces and ketchup can aggravate reflux disease.

Cocoa: There are compounds in chocolate that have the potential to relax the lower esophageal sphincter (LES), reopening the esophagus to stomach acid.

Mint: Peppermint and spearmint are two types of mint that can relax the LES and exacerbate symptoms of acid reflux. This also holds true for sweets and gum with a mint taste.

Hot Foods: Foods that are extremely seasoned or spicy might irritate the esophagus and cause reflux. Choose tastier seasonings.

fatty and fried foods: meals high in fat, particularly fried meals, can slow down the emptying of the stomach and raise the risk of acid reflux.

Carbonated Drinks: Carbonated beverages, such as sodas, have the potential to increase reflux and pressure in the digestive tract by allowing more air to enter it.

Coffee and Other Caffeinated Drinks: Because caffeine relaxes the LES, stomach acid can more easily reflux back into the esophagus. Reduce or give up coffee-based beverages.

Spirits: Alcohol can cause the LES to relax and increase the production of stomach acid. Alcohol intake can be minimized or avoided to help control GERD symptoms.

Highly Manipulated Foods: Acid reflux may be exacerbated by processed and packaged meals, which are frequently heavy in chemicals and preservatives. Choose unprocessed or lightly processed foods.

## Success Advice:
### The Key Is Moderation:

Be mindful of portion sizes and refrain from overindulging, since larger meals may result in increased stomach strain.

When to Eat: To give the stomach time to empty, give yourself at least two to three hours between meals and bedtime.

Maintain Hydration: To keep hydrated, sip water throughout the day, but try not to consume too much during meals.

Maintain a Food Diary: Keep a food journal and record any symptoms you have. Finding trigger foods and patterns might be aided by this.

Speak with a Medical Professional:

Seek help from a healthcare provider for individualized advice and maybe additional assessment if symptoms worsen or continue.

Through the use of these dietary recommendations, people may customize their eating patterns to effectively manage acid reflux. It's critical to understand that everyone has different tolerances, and that alterations may be required depending on how each person reacts to particular meals. Always seek the opinion of a medical practitioner to rule out any underlying issues and to receive specific recommendations.

# CHAPTER 3

## Benefits of Following an Acid Reflux Diet

There are several advantages to following an acid reflux diet, including symptom alleviation and improved digestive health in general. The following are the main advantages of an acid reflux diet:

1. Decreased Heartburn and Regurgitation: One of the main advantages of an acid reflux diet is a notable decrease in the reflux's signature symptoms, heartburn and regurgitation. Through conscious dietary choices and avoidance of trigger foods, people can reduce the frequency and intensity of these painful experiences.

2. Better Sleep: When lying down, acid reflux symptoms can get worse, which interferes with getting a good night's sleep. A diet that reduces acid reflux, particularly when big meals are avoided just before bed, can help with better quality sleep. Reflux symptoms throughout the night might be further relieved by raising the head of the bed.

3. Preventing Esophageal Damage: Acid reflux disease (GERD) can result in erosive esophagitis, an inflammatory disorder that damages the esophagus due to stomach acid. People can reduce their chance of acquiring esophageal issues and facilitate the recovery of any damage already done by following an acid reflux diet.

4. Weight Control: Resolving acid reflux requires maintaining a healthy weight. Consuming nutrient-dense, lower-calorie meals is encouraged by an acid reflux diet, which helps with weight management. Overweight, particularly in the abdominal area, might exacerbate reflux symptoms by raising intra-abdominal pressure.

5. Improved Digestive Comfort: The focus of an acid reflux diet is on foods that are simple to digest and don't cause discomfort to the digestive system as a whole. Choosing foods that are easy on the digestive system can help people lessen the chance that their stomach contents will reflux back into their esophagus.

6. Reduced Complications: Prolonged acid reflux can cause more severe ailments including Barrett's esophagus, a precancerous alteration in the esophageal lining. An acid reflux diet helps reduce difficulties and provides a preventive measure against more serious health problems.

7. Enhanced Nutrient Absorption: Symptoms of acid reflux disease may make it more difficult for the body to absorb vital nutrients. Through dietary management of reflux, people can enhance their absorption of nutrients, hence promoting general health and wellness.

8. Better Quality of Life: Having acid reflux on a regular basis can have a major negative influence on a person's quality of life. Following an acid reflux diet helps people feel less affected by their symptoms, which makes it easier and more enjoyable for them to participate in everyday activities, social gatherings, and meals.

9. Tailored Approach: There is no one-size-fits-all acid reflux diet. It enables people to identify their

own triggers and adjust their eating patterns accordingly. Individuals are empowered to make decisions that are tailored to their unique requirements by keeping a diet log and identifying patterns of symptoms.

10. Long-Term Health Benefits: An acid reflux diet helps to maintain long-term health in addition to alleviating short-term symptoms. People can lower their chance of developing other lifestyle-related illnesses including obesity, diabetes, and cardiovascular problems by adopting good eating habits.

11. Less Dependency on Medications: Many people find that following an acid reflux diet reduces their need for drugs like proton pump inhibitors, H2 blockers, and antacids. For people who are worried about these drugs' possible long-term negative effects, this can be very helpful.

In summary, adhering to an acid reflux diet is a comprehensive strategy for maintaining digestive health that goes beyond treating symptoms. People can alleviate discomfort, avoid difficulties, and enhance their general health by making thoughtful eating choices. A licensed dietitian or other healthcare expert can offer individualized advice, ensuring that dietary modifications support long-term health advantages and are in line with individual needs.

## How To Follow This Acid Reflux Diet

Making thoughtful and educated decisions is part of adhering to an acid reflux diet in order to reduce symptoms and encourage digestive comfort. This is a thorough guide on how to start and maintain an acid reflux diet:

1. Educate Yourself: Start by being familiar with the fundamentals of an acid reflux diet. Learn about your trigger foods, which typically include chocolate, mint, citrus fruits, tomatoes, spicy meals, and fatty or fried foods. Knowing these triggers is essential to choose a diet that works for you.

2. Maintain a Food Journal: Record the foods you eat each day and any symptoms you encounter. By identifying certain triggers and trends, this notebook can help manage acid reflux in a more individualized and efficient manner.

3. Select Fruits with Low Acidity: Go for non-citrus fruits like bananas, apples, and pears. These fruits are not as likely to make symptoms of acid reflux worse.

4. Choose Non-Acidic veggies: Add a range of veggies to your diet, but concentrate on things like potatoes, cauliflower, broccoli, and green leafy vegetables. To preserve the nutritious content of veggies, steam or sauté them gently.

5. Lean Proteins: Select lean meats, fish, and poultry as your lean protein sources. It is better to grill, bake, or simmer these proteins instead of frying them.

6. Use Whole Grains: Choose whole grains such as quinoa, brown rice, and oatmeal. Because of the fiber in these grains, digestion is aided and general digestive health is promoted.

7. Minimize or Steer Clear of Dairy: Opt for fat-free or low-fat dairy products. Keep an eye on your dairy tolerance because some people may discover that particular dairy products aggravate symptoms of acid reflux.

8. Mindful Eating: Engage in mindful eating by giving your meal a good chew and enjoying every taste. A bigger meal can put more strain on the

stomach and raise the risk of acid reflux, so try not to overeat.

9. Healthy Fats: Include foods like avocados, almonds, and olive oil in your diet as sources of healthy fats. Unlike trans or saturated fats, these fats are less prone to cause acid reflux.

10. Herbs and Spices: To improve flavor without adding too much acidity, use mild herbs and spices like fennel, ginger, and oregano. Steer clear of using too many strong spices since they might irritate the esophagus.

11. Non-Caffeinated Drinks: Sip herbal teas, water, and liquids without flavors of mint or citrus. Drink plenty of water throughout the day, but refrain from consuming too much during meals.

12. Ginger: Add some ginger to your meals. Ginger is well-known for its anti-inflammatory qualities and ability to calm the digestive system, whether it is used as a spice or in tea.

13. Timing of Meals: Give yourself at least two or three hours between meals and going to bed. This lowers the chance of acid reflux during periods of inactivity by giving the stomach time to empty.

14. Steer Clear of Trigger items: Recognize and cut out trigger items from your diet. If particular foods are known to trigger symptoms on a regular basis, it is best to eliminate or reduce their intake.

15. Raise the Head of the Bed: You should raise the head of your bed by six to eight inches if you have reflux at night. By doing this, you may be able to stop the reflux of stomach acid into your esophagus at night.

16. Restrict or Steer clear of Alcohol and Caffeine: These substances have the ability to relax the lower esophageal sphincter (LES), which can exacerbate acid reflux. Reduce or cut out these foods from your diet.

17. Give Up Smoking: If you smoke, think about giving it up. Smoking impairs the LES and

increases the risk of acid reflux developing or getting worse.

18. Consistent Exercise: – Take part in consistent physical exercise. Exercise can improve gut health, help control weight, and enhance general health.

19. Speak with a Medical Expert: Seek advice from a healthcare provider if symptoms worsen or continue. If required, they can do diagnostic testing, offer specialized counsel, and create a treatment plan that is tailored to your individual requirements.

Adopting an acid reflux diet is a proactive, self-empowering strategy for symptom management and digestive health promotion. It entails selecting meals carefully, developing mindful eating practices, and identifying and avoiding triggers. You may take charge of your nutrition and enhance your general quality of life by adopting these recommendations into your everyday routine. To verify that dietary modifications are in line with your specific health needs, always seek the counsel of a healthcare practitioner.

## Complications If the Right Diet Isn't Adopted.

Beyond the occasional heartburn, there are a number of problems that can arise from not following an acid reflux diet. The esophagus and general health may suffer greatly as a result of failing to control acid reflux through dietary decisions. The following are possible side effects of not following a suitable diet for acid reflux:

1. Esophagitis: An inflammation of the esophagus, esophagitis is one of the main consequences of untreated acid reflux. Constant contact to stomach acid can cause irritation, redness, and swelling of the esophageal lining, which in turn can develop to esophagitis.

2. Strictures of the Esophagus:

Prolonged esophageal inflammation can cause scar tissue to grow, which can result in the development of strictures or constricted regions. Esophageal strictures can make swallowing difficult, and their relief may need medical attention.

The development of Barrett's esophagus, a disorder in which the normal lining of the esophagus is replaced by tissue that mimics the lining of the intestine, is another risk factor associated with chronic acid reflux. There is a higher chance of esophageal cancer linked to this modification.

4. Esophageal Cancer: Untreated acid reflux, particularly when compounded by Barrett's esophagus, raises the chance of developing esophageal cancer, while it is a very uncommon condition. For those with Barrett's esophagus, ongoing monitoring and treatment are essential to halting the disease's development into cancer.

5. Respiratory Complications: Recurrent pneumonia, asthma, and persistent cough are among the respiratory conditions that can result from stomach acid flowing back into the esophagus and into the lungs. These issues have the potential to worsen breathing problems and impair respiratory health in general.

6. Dental Problems: Tooth enamel that is frequently exposed to stomach acid may experience erosion, corrosion, and sensitivity. Acid reflux left untreated might lead to oral health issues that need for dental work.

7. Prolonged Sore Throat and Hoarseness: Prolonged sore throat and hoarseness may be brought on by the discomfort that acid reflux causes. Stomach acid exposure over time can cause vocal cord injury and permanent voice abnormalities.

8. Sleep disturbances: If left untreated, acid reflux frequently gets worse at night, which throws off sleep cycles. Fatigue, irritation, and a lowered sense of general wellbeing can all be caused by insomnia and poor sleep quality.

9. Impaired Nutrient Absorption: Nutritional deficits can result from chronic acid reflux's interference with the body's ability to absorb vital nutrients. Over time, a number of health problems

may be attributed to inadequate absorption of vitamins and minerals.

10. Decreased Quality of Life: Acid reflux may have a major negative influence on a person's quality of life if left untreated. Prolonged symptoms, discomfort, and worry about future developments can cause worry, tension, and a lowered feeling of general wellbeing.

11. Increased Reliance on Medications: People with untreated acid reflux may become too dependent on drugs like antacids, H2 blockers, or proton pump inhibitors if they don't make dietary and lifestyle modifications. The prolonged usage of these drugs may come with hazards and adverse consequences.

12. Avoiding Trigger Foods: People may continue eating trigger foods that worsen their symptoms if they are unaware of them and do not follow an acid reflux diet. This may exacerbate the pain cycle and hasten the development of problems.

13. Limited Treatment Options: The efficacy of various treatments for acid reflux may be hampered

if the proper diet is not followed. If dietary changes are not included in the overall therapy plan, medications and surgical procedures may not be as effective.

Finally, ignoring the need to follow an acid reflux diet can lead to a host of issues that go far beyond the occasional soreness. The effects, which range from esophageal inflammation to an elevated risk of esophageal cancer, highlight the significance of proactive treatment through food and lifestyle choices. To avoid potential issues and support long-term digestive health, it is imperative that people with acid reflux symptoms seek advice from healthcare specialists, adopt suitable dietary adjustments, and implement lifestyle changes.

# CHAPTER 4

## Breakfast Recipes

Here are ten breakfast dishes that are acid reflux-friendly, along with the ingredients and cooking techniques for each:

## Banana and Almond Oatmeal:
### Ingredients:

- 1/2 cup rolled oats
- One ripe banana, cut.
- One tablespoon of finely chopped almonds
- One tsp honey

### Preparation:

1. Follow the directions on the package to cook the oats.
2. Add chopped almonds, banana slices, and a honey drizzle over top.

## Greek Yogurt Parfait:
- Contains 1 cup of plain Greek yogurt as an ingredient.
- Half a cup of low-fat granola

- ½ cup of mixed berries, including raspberries, blueberries, and strawberries

**Preparation**

1. Arrange Greek yogurt, granola, and mixed berries in a glass or dish.
2. After layering again, serve.

## Egg and Spinach Scramble:

- Add 2 beaten eggs to the mixture.
- One cup finely chopped fresh spinach and one tablespoon of optional feta cheese
- To taste, add salt and pepper.

**Preparation:**

1. Cook chopped spinach in a skillet until it wilts.
2. Add the feta cheese, salt, pepper, and beaten eggs. Eggs should be scrambled until done.

## Whole Grain Toast with Avocado:

- Contains two pieces of toasted whole grain bread.
- 1/2 mashed, ripe avocado

- Sliced cherry tomatoes
- Chia seed sprinkle (optional)

**Preparation**

1. Toast the pieces of whole grain bread as preparation.
2. Toast is slathered with mashed avocado, then chia seeds and cherry tomato slices are added.

## Smoothie Bowl:

- Compostable berries: 1 cup, frozen
- half a banana
- half a cup of Greek yogurt, plain
- One spoonful of honey

**Preparation**

1. To prepare, blend Greek yogurt, frozen berries, and banana until smooth.
2. Transfer to a bowl and top with honey. If preferred, sprinkle more granola or fruit over top.

## Breakfast Bowl with Quinoa:
**Ingredients:**

- Half a cup of cooked quinoa
- Slicing 1/4 cup of almonds
- Half a cup of peaches, sliced
- One spoonful of honey

**Preparation:**

1. In a bowl, mix cooked quinoa, sliced peaches, and sliced almonds.
2. Pour honey over it and stir thoroughly.

## Pancakes made with Buckwheat:
**Ingredients**

- Half a cup of buckwheat flour
- half a cup of almond milk
- One egg

**Preparation**

- One-half tsp baking powder
1. To prepare, combine buckwheat flour, egg, almond milk, and baking powder in a bowl.

2. To cook, pour onto a hot griddle or pancake pan.

## Pineapple and Cottage Cheese Bowl:
**Ingredients:**

- half a cup of cottage cheese without fat
- half a cup of raw pineapple pieces
- One tablespoon of coconut shreds

**Preparation**

1. To prepare, combine pineapple chunks and cottage cheese in a bowl.
2. Add some shredded coconut on top.

## Almond Butter and Banana Wrap:
**Ingredients**

- One whole wheat tortilla as an ingredient
- Two tsp almond butter
- One banana, cut into slices

**Preparation**

1. To prepare, spread the whole wheat tortilla with almond butter.

2. After adding the sliced banana, wrap it.

## Chia Seed Pudding:
### Ingredients

- Two tsp chia seeds - half a cup almond milk
- Half a teaspoon of essence from vanilla
- Fresh berries to garnish with Getting ready:

### Preparation

1. In a container, combine chia seeds, almond milk, and vanilla essence.
2. Give it a good stir, then chill for the night.
3. Before serving, place some fresh berries on top.

These breakfast foods are appropriate for those who manage acid reflux since they are meant to be easy on the digestive system. Depending on dietary requirements and personal tastes, modify ingredient and quantity quantities.

# CHAPTER 5

## Lunch Recipes

Here are ten lunch dishes that are acid reflux-friendly, complete with ingredients and preparation instructions:

## Grilled Chicken Salad:

- Made using grilled chicken breast as an ingredient
- mixed greens (spinach and lettuce)
- Cherry tomatoes, cucumber slices, and balsamic vinegar and olive oil for dressing

### Preparation

1. Prepare by slicing and grilling the chicken breast.
2. Toss with cucumber, cherry tomatoes, and mixed greens. Add grilled chicken on top and drizzle with balsamic vinegar and olive oil.

## Stir-Fry with Quinoa and Vegetables:

**Ingredients:**

- cooked quinoa
- mixed veggies, including carrots, broccoli, and bell peppers
- Grilled chicken or tofu (optional)
- Sodium-free soy sauce

**Preparation**

1. Prepare the veggies by pan-frying them until they become soft.
2. Add grilled chicken or tofu along with the cooked quinoa. Add low-sodium soy sauce and stir.

## Foil Pack of Salmon and Asparagus:
**Ingredients:**

- Salmon fillet
- spears of asparagus
- Slices of lemon
- Olive oil

**Preparation**

1. Salmon fillet should be prepared by placing it on foil.
2. Place the asparagus next to the salmon, top with slices of lemon, and dress with olive oil. After sealing the foil, bake.
3. Millet Bowl with Roasted Vegetables:

## Millet should be cooked.

- roasted veggies, such as bell peppers, cherry tomatoes, and zucchini
- Feta cheese, if desired
- Lemon dressing with olive oil

### Preparation

1. Prepare by combining roasted veggies and cooked millet.
2. Add feta cheese on top and drizzle with lemon and olive oil.

## Avocado and Turkey Wrap:
### Ingredients:

- Sliced turkey
- wrap made with whole wheat

Avocado and thinly sliced spinach

**Preparation**

1. Arrange the turkey slices on a wrap made entirely of whole wheat.
2. Fold in the sliced avocado and spinach leaves.

# Quinoa Chili with Vegetables:
**Ingredients:**

- cooked quinoa
- Black beans, pinto beans, and kidney beans
- chopped tomatoes
- Cumin and chili powder

**Preparation**

1. To prepare, mix cooked quinoa with diced tomatoes, beans, and seasonings.
2. Once the flavors have blended, simmer and serve with desired toppings.

# Stir-fried Shrimp and Vegetables:
**Ingredients:**

- Peeled and deveined shrimp
- florets of broccoli
- Snap peas
- Ginger and garlic
- teriyaki sauce with low sodium

**Preparation**

1. Prepare by pan-sautéing shrimp, snap peas, broccoli, garlic, and ginger.
2. After adding the low-sodium teriyaki sauce, stir everything until it is well cooked.

## Spinach and Mushroom Frittata:
### Ingredients:

- Eggs
- Sliced mushrooms
- fresh spinach
- Feta cheese

**Preparation**

1. To prepare, beat the eggs and transfer them onto a pan.

2. Add the feta cheese, mushrooms, and fresh spinach. Bake until solidified.

## Lentil and Veggie Soup:
- Contains either brown or green lentils as an ingredient.
- Celery, onion, and carrots
- Reduced-sodium vegetable stock
- Spinach leaves

**Preparation**

1. Prepare the lentils and veggies by cooking them in a vegetable broth low in sodium.
2. Serve with spinach leaves added right before.

Because these lunch meals are meant to be easy on the digestive system, even individuals who manage acid reflux may enjoy them. Depending on dietary requirements and personal tastes, modify ingredient and quantity quantities.

# CHAPTER 6

## Dinner Recipes
## Baked Salmon with Dill and Lemon:
### Ingredients:

- Fillets of salmon
- Slices of lemon
- new dill
- Olive oil

### Preparation

1. Salmon fillets should be prepared by preheating the oven and putting them on a baking pan.
2. Add a sprinkle of olive oil, lemon slices, and fresh dill on top. Bake the fish until it's done.

## Quinoa Stuffed Bell Peppers:
### Ingredients:

- half a bell pepper, cooked Quinoa
- Diced tomatoes, corn, and black beans
- For seasoning, use paprika and cumin.

**Preparation**

1. Prepare the quinoa by combining it with chopped tomatoes, black beans, and corn.
2. Add paprika and cumin for seasoning. Bake the stuffed bell peppers until they are soft.

## Sweet potato wedges with grilled turkey burger:
**Ingredients:**

- Ground turkey
- Burger buns made entirely of wheat
- Cut the sweet potatoes into wedges.
- To season, use rosemary and olive oil.

**Preparation**

1. Prepare by shaping ground turkey into patties and cooking on a grill.
2. Sweet potato wedges should be tossed with rosemary and olive oil before baking till brown.

## Stir-fried Brown Rice for Veggies:
**Ingredients:**

- Cooked brown rice
- Various veggies, including bell peppers, carrots, and broccoli
- Tempeh or tofu
- Sodium-free soy sauce

**Preparation:**

1. Stir-fry various veggies along with tempeh or tofu.
2. Mix in the cooked brown rice and low-sodium soy sauce.

## Vegetable and Chicken Skewers:
**Ingredients:**

- Cubes of chicken breast
- Bell peppers, cherry tomatoes, and zucchini
- Herbs and olive oil for marinating

**Preparation**

1. Prepare the ingredients by marinating veggies and chicken cubes in olive oil and seasonings.

2. After the chicken is threaded onto skewers, grill until done.

## Eggplant and Tomato Bake:
**Ingredients:**

- sliced mozzarella cheese, sliced tomatoes, and eggplant
- fresh leaves of basil

**Preparation**

1. Steps to follow: Arrange tomatoes and sliced eggplant in a baking dish.
2. Add fresh basil and mozzarella cheese on top. Bake till frothy.

## Turkey Bolognese with Squash:
**Ingredients:**

- spaghetti squash
- Turkey on the ground
- Low-acid tomato sauce
- Italian herbs and garlic for flavoring

**Preparation**

1. To prepare, roast the spaghetti squash until it becomes soft, then scrape it into strands.
2. Add tomato sauce, garlic, and Italian herbs after cooking ground turkey. Put on top of spaghetti squash.

## Stir-fried cauliflower rice:
**Ingredients:**

- Chicken or shrimp?
- Vegetable mixture (peas, carrots, corn)
- teriyaki sauce with low sodium

**Preparation**

1. Prepare by stirring-frying mixed veggies, shrimp, or chicken, and cauliflower rice.
2. Stir in low-sodium teriyaki sauce and heat thoroughly.

## Grilled chicken salad with lemon herbs:
**Ingredients:**

- Grilled chicken breast
- mixed greens (spinach, arugula)
- Red onion, cucumber, and cherry tomatoes

- Dressing with lemon vinaigrette

**Preparation**

1. Prepare by grilling and slicing a chicken breast.
2. Toss with red onion, cucumber, cherry tomatoes, and mixed greens. Add some grilled chicken on top and pour some lemon vinaigrette over it.

## Baked cod with mashed sweet potatoes:
**Ingredients**

1. Cod fillets, sliced and peeled sweet potatoes, and Greek yogurt
2. Garnish with fresh parsley.
3. Seared cod fillets should be flaky.

**Preparation**

To make sweet potatoes creamier, boil and mash them with Greek yogurt. Garnish fish with fresh parsley and serve it over mashed sweet potatoes.

These meal dishes are ideal for those who manage acid reflux since they are designed to be easy on the digestive system. Depending on dietary requirements and personal tastes, modify ingredient and quantity quantities.

# CONCLUSION

To sum up, adopting an acid reflux diet is a proactive and powerful strategy to control symptoms, improve digestive health, and avert future issues. A conscious eating style, avoiding triggers, and cautious food selection all play a part in leading a lifetime free from acid reflux pain. People can lower the risk of problems including esophagitis, strictures, and even esophageal cancer by promoting healing and healing-promoting foods such as lean proteins, healthy grains, and a variety of fruits and vegetables.

Furthermore, the acid reflux diet offers a comprehensive strategy for general wellbeing, going beyond the treatment of symptoms. Among the many advantages of following this food plan are better sleep, increased nutritional absorption, and less dependency on drugs. Because the diet is adaptable, people may customize it to meet their own requirements by recognizing and avoiding certain triggers by using tools like food journals.

As you set out on this path to improved digestive health, keep in mind that minor adjustments can have a big impact. Encourage yourself by imagining a life where discomfort is minimized, energy is maximized, and overall wellbeing is elevated. You are investing in your health and well-being when you stick to this acid reflux diet. Seize the chance to enjoy meals that provide nourishment to your body and ease intestinal distress. You are creating a future free from acid reflux's limitations and long-lasting advantages with every deliberate decision you make. The decisions you make today will determine the path to intestinal harmony, and your well-being is worth the effort. Cheers to a happier, healthier you!

# Contact Us

**Dear Reader,**

**If you have any questions, need further clarification, or require assistance with any aspect of the book, please do not hesitate to reach out to me. I am more than happy to provide additional insights, address your queries, or simply engage in a meaningful discussion.**

**Feel free to contact me at: IsabelleHartleyBooks@gmail.com. Your feedback and inquiries are always welcome.**

# FREE 30 DAYS MEAL PLANNER

FREE 30Days Meal Planner, a priceless extra to get you started on the path to a more organized and healthy living. This meticulously curated planner is made to make meal planning easier, save you time, and help you meet your nutritional objectives. Prepare to enjoy the advantages of this wonderful resource! Scan the QR Code below now.

www.ingramcontent.com/pod-product-compliance
Lightning Source LLC
Chambersburg PA
CBHW062249290526
45794CB00006B/2468